The Ebola Survival Manual

A collection of tips, strategies, and
supply lists from some of the world's
best preparedness professionals

This collaboration would not be possible without the generosity of Tess Pennington, Daisy Luther, Lizzie Bennett, Lily Dane, Lisa Egan and Mac Slavo

Ebola.

Even the name of the virus conjures up mental images of a gruesome, agonizing, bloody death.

Anyone who has scanned the news headlines lately has, at the very least, an inkling that a horrible disease is on the loose. It's anyone's best guess how soon this becomes a pandemic on American soil. While the Center for Disease Control and the World Health Organization have both expressed serious concerns that we are on the brink of disaster, border enforcement agencies seem blithely unconcerned.

It's really up to you to protect your family. This is a collection of some of the best information in the preparedness community to help keep you and your family safe throughout this potential pandemic.

Checklists are provided at the end of the book to help you gather the necessary supplies quickly and efficiently.

Part One:

Is Ebola Really a Threat?

Hospitals Prep for Ebola Outbreak: Cases May Exceed 100,000 by December: "The Numbers Are Really Scary"

By Mac Slavo

Though news on the Ebola virus has been muted since two American health care workers were admitted to U.S.-based facilities last month, the deadly contagion continues to spread. According to the World Health Organization more than 40% of all Ebola cases[1] thus far have occurred in just the last three months, suggesting that the virus is continuing to build steam.

Physicist Alessandro Vespignani of Northeastern University in Boston is one of several researchers trying to figure out how far Ebola may spread and how many people around the world could be affected. Based on his findings, there will be 10,000 cases by

---

[1] http://online.wsj.com/articles/ebola-virus-outbreak-could-hit-20-000-within-nine-months-warns-who-1409226146

4

September of this year and it only gets worse from there.

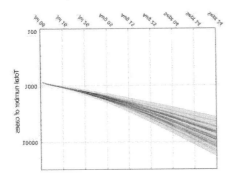

(A model created by Alessandro Vespignani and his colleagues suggests that, at its current spread, Ebola may infect up to 10,000 people by September 24. Other models suggest up to 100,000 infected globally by December of this year. The shaded area is the variability range.)

*Extrapolating existing trends, the number of the sick and dying mounts rapidly from the current toll—more than 3000 cases and 1500 deaths—to around 10,000 cases by September 24, and hundreds of thousands in the months after that. **"The numbers are really scary,"** he says—although he stresses that the model assumes control efforts aren't stepped up. **"We all hope to see this NOT*** *happening," Vespignani writes in an e-mail.*

...

*Vespignani is not the only one trying to predict how the unprecedented outbreak will progress. Last week, the World Health Organization (WHO) estimated that the number of cases could ultimately exceed 20,000. And scientists across the world are scrambling to create computer models that accurately describe the spread of the deadly virus. Not all of them look quite as bleak as Vespignani's. But the modelers all agree that **current efforts to control the epidemic are <u>not enough</u> to stop the deadly pathogen in its tracks.***

...

"If the epidemic in Liberia were to continue in this way until the 1st of December, the cumulative number of cases would exceed 100,000," *predicts Althaus. Such long-term forecasts are error-prone, he acknowledges.*

...

*Vespignani has analyzed the likelihood that Ebola will spread to other countries. Using data on millions of air travelers and commuters, as well as mobility patterns based on data from censuses and mobile devices, he has built a model of the world, into which he can introduce Ebola and then run hundreds of thousands of simulations. In general, the chance of further spread beyond West Africa is small, Vespignani says, but **the risk grows with the scale of the epidemic.***

Ghana, the United Kingdom, and the United States are among the countries most likely to have an introduced case, according to the model.

Source: Science Mag[2] and WHO

Though researchers and officials hope that this is "not happening," the fact is that Ebola spread has only increased since it was first identified earlier this year. And now it is spreading to densely populated African cities like Lagos, Nigeria.

---

[2] http://news.sciencemag.org/health/2014/08/disease-modelers-project-rapidly-rising-toll-ebola

The Centers for Disease Control and US-based hospitals maintain that the likelihood of Ebola spreading to the United States remains "extremely low," but that hasn't stopped them from preparing infection control protocols because of the extremely high fatality rates associated with those who contract the virus.

Hospitals throughout Southern California are preparing for potential Ebola cases, even as they seek to reassure patients and health care workers that the risk is very low.

…

Public health officials say with the right isolation and infection control procedures, all hospitals could safely handle a patient with Ebola without exposing staff or other patients.

"We have the infrastructure anyway because we see these things on a daily basis. We see tuberculosis, influenza, potentially measles, and whooping cough," said Dr. Zachary Rubin, medical director of clinical epidemiology and infection prevention at UCLA. "Even though Ebola is in the news, this is something we do day in and day out."

The CDC's Ebola recommendations for hospitals include an array of measures such as private rooms for patients, protective coverings for staff, and limiting use of needles as much as possible to prevent transmission.

...

"In the context of overall diseases, the likelihood of Ebola even coming to the U.S. or to UCI Medical Center is so extremely low, we just don't expect it to happen," Gohil said.

"However, the fatalities are so high and the possibility of travel in the global context is just enough that we have to prepare. One of the reasons you want to prepare is to reassure your staff and your patients that it's perfectly handleable."

Public health officials say with the right isolation and infection control procedures, all hospitals could safely handle a patient with Ebola without exposing staff or other patients.

Source: Los Angeles Register[3]

Experts say the virus doesn't spread like the flu or measles because it is not airborne. However, there are some indications that current strain of the Ebola virus may be mutating. Last month a warning issued by the

---

[3] http://www.losangelesregister.com/articles/ebola-604191-patient-infection.html

CDC[4] claimed that infectious Ebola materials could be spread through the air.

The advisory urges airline staff to provide surgical masks to potential Ebola victims in order "to reduce the number of droplets expelled into the air by talking, sneezing, or coughing."

The CDC is also directing airline cleaning personnel to, "not use compressed air, which might spread infectious material through the air." (Emphasis mine).

The CDC's concern about the Ebola virus being spread via the air is understandable in light of a 2012 experiment conducted by Canadian scientists[5] which proved that, "the Ebola virus could be transmitted by air between species."

At this time it is too early to tell if efforts by health officials in Africa, Europe and the USA will be effective in stopping the virus. All indications suggest it will continue to spread, just as it has for nearly a year.

The disease models, which are based on population density and mobility patterns,

---

[4] http://www.thedailysheeple.com/its-airborne-cdc-warns-of-infectious-material-through-the-air_082014
[5] http://www.bbc.com/news/science-environment-20341423

show that it is only a matter of time before an infection is identified in the United States.

In the event that a single person in the Western hemisphere acquires it, then chances are there will be more.

Hospitals in the United States may be preparing isolation protocols, but what about Mexico, where the southern border has been left completely exposed? With cramped quarters on trains and trucks carrying hundreds or thousands of migrants, and unsanitary conditions, it is quite possible that a single infected individual could pass the virus on to scores of others, who in turn would disperse to various cities as soon as they reached US-soil.

And that doesn't even include the millions of travelers arriving and departing at US airports from coast to coast on a daily basis.

The CDC and US healthcare officials may think they can control it, but all such efforts around the world have failed thus far.

Moreover, should an Ebola outbreak occur in the United States, the panic it will cause may exceed what we saw during the H1N1 flu scare several years ago. Over 25% of American adults fear that the virus could spread to a family member or close friend because of its high fatality rate. This suggests that any indication of contagion on US shores will lead to a run on medical supplies once the virus becomes reality here at home.

The healthcare system could be overwhelmed and medical supplies could feel a serious crunch as panicked Americans race to acquire everything from WHO recommended N-100 masks to protective body suits.

Ebola Outbreak is "Spiraling Out of Control"

By Lily Dane

As the largest Ebola outbreak in world history rages on, more questions and concerns about containing the virus are being raised.

During a briefing yesterday[6], Dr. Thomas Frieden, director of the Centers for Disease Control and Prevention (CDC), said that the outbreak in West Africa is "spiraling out of control". He said that the international community "can control it, if we act now, but the window of opportunity is closing."

As of August 28, Ebola has infected 3,069 people and caused 1,552 deaths, according to the CDC.[7]

Last Thursday, the World Health Organization (WHO) reported[8]that nearly 40% of those cases occurred within the last three weeks.

---

[6] http://www.businessinsider.com/cdc-director-tom-frieden-ebola-update-2014-9
[7] http://www.cdc.gov/vhf/ebola/outbreaks/guinea/
[8]
http://www.who.int/mediacentre/news/releases/2014/ebola-roadmap/en/

The WHO also warned that this outbreak could eventually infect more than 20,000 people.

Dr. Bruce Aylward, WHO's assistant director-general for emergency operations, said[9] part of the problem is that the outbreak is occurring in large cities and broad sections of the affected countries:

"What we are seeing today, in contrast to previous Ebola outbreaks: multiple hotspots within these countries — not a single, remote forested area, the kind of environments that have been tackled in the past. And then not multiple hotspots within one country, but international disease.

This far outstrips any historic Ebola outbreak in numbers. The largest outbreak in the past was about 400 cases."

Yesterday, the international group Doctors Without Borders warned that the world is losing the battle against Ebola and that treatment centers in West Africa have been "reduced to places where people go to die alone", reports the AP[10]:

---

[9] http://www.webmd.com/news/20140828/ebola-outbreak-could-infect-20000-people-un-says
[10] http://www.aol.com/article/2014/09/03/doctors-without-borders-world-is-losing-the-battle-against-

Doctors Without Borders, which has treated more than 1,000 Ebola patients in West Africa since March, is completely overwhelmed by the disease, said Joanne Liu, the organization's president. She called on other countries to contribute civilian and military medical personnel familiar with biological disasters.

"Six months into the worst Ebola epidemic in history, the world is losing the battle to contain it," Liu said at a U.N. forum on the outbreak. "Ebola treatment centers are reduced to places where people go to die alone, where little more than palliative care is offered."

In Sierra Leone, she said, infectious bodies are rotting in the streets. Liberia had to build a new crematorium instead of new Ebola care centers.

Liu said[11] the situation is dire in parts of West Africa, and spoke of overwhelmed isolation centers, riots breaking out over controversial quarantines, infected bodies lying in the

---

ebo/20956214/?icid=maing-grid7%7Cmaing8%7Cdl10%7Csec1_lnk3%26pLid%3D524082
[11]http://www.washingtonpost.com/news/to-your-health/wp/2014/09/02/another-u-s-doctor-in-liberia-tests-positive-for-ebola/

streets, medical workers dying in shocking numbers, and entire health systems crumbling.

Dr. Daniel Bausch, a WHO-sponsored doctor who is working in Sierra Leone, described conditions to Business Insider[12]:

"You have a very dangerous virus in three of the countries in the world that are least equipped to deal with it. The scale of this outbreak has just outstripped the resources. That's why it's become so big.

You have people saying they don't have food, they don't have water, they need their IV replaced — and you're trying to do all of that. I need to wash my hands before I see the patients, and there might be no running water. There [is sometimes] no soap, no clean needles."

Liu said the only way the outbreak can be contained is if governments send in biohazard teams and equipment.

From The Guardian[13]:

---

[12] http://www.businessinsider.com/how-ebola-is-spread-and-transmitted-2014-8

[13] http://www.theguardian.com/society/2014/sep/02/ebola-outbreak-call-send-m

"Many of the member states represented here today have invested heavily in biological threat response," she said at the UN. *"You have a political and humanitarian responsibility to immediately utilise these capabilities in Ebola-affected countries.*

"To curb the epidemic, it is imperative that states immediately deploy civilian and military assets with expertise in biohazard containment. I call upon you to dispatch your disaster response teams, backed by the full weight of your logistical capabilities. This should be done in close collaboration with the affected countries. Without this deployment, we will never get the epidemic under control."

She [Liu] said, there must be a change of approach by affected countries. "Coercive measures, such as laws criminalizing the failure to report suspected cases, and forced quarantines, are driving people underground.

"This is leading to the concealment of cases, and is pushing the sick away from health systems. These measures have only served to breed fear and unrest, rather than contain the virus."

Food shortages are also a threat, as restrictions on trade and movement are in place in the Ebola-hit countries.

A disturbing video of a patient leaving quarantine to find food at a market in Monrovia, Liberia, demonstrates the fear and desperation people are experiencing there. The video shows the man being chased and caught by doctors while onlookers watch. A woman in the video says that Ebola patients are not being fed:

"The patients are hungry, they are starving. No food, no water. The government need to do more," she said.

Meanwhile, another physician from the U.S. has tested positive for Ebola, reports The Washington Post[14]:

> *The unnamed missionary doctor was treating obstetrics patients at the organization's ELWA hospital in Monrovia, Liberia, and was not working with Ebola patients in the facility's isolation unit, which is separate from the main hospital, according to a news*

---

[14] http://www.washingtonpost.com/news/to-your-health/wp/2014/09/02/another-u-s-doctor-in-liberia-tests-positive-for-ebola/

release from the organization. He isolated himself immediately upon developing symptoms and has been transferred to the Ebola isolation unit.

What Is Not Being Said Publicly: Ebola Virus's Hyper-Evolution is Unprecedented… Could Go Airborne

By Mac Slavo

The last several months have led to much confusion about the spread of the Ebola virus. Health officials and governments first denied that a serious threat existed and took no significant action to prevent its spread outside of West Africa. Then, after it had made its way to six different countries in the region, officials at the World Health Organization and the U.S. Centers for Disease Control started to panic. Apathy gave way to the real fear that we were facing a virus on a whole different scale than ever before.

At its current rate, some mathematical models show that the virus could infect anywhere from 20,000 to 100,000 people[15] by the end of the year, with over 4,000 people worldwide having been infected thus far. About 2,300

---

[15] http://www.shtfplan.com/headline-news/u-s-hospitals-prep-for-ebola-outbreak-cases-may-exceed-100000-by-december-the-numbers-are-really-scary_09012014

people, over 50% of those who have contracted it, have died.

Although the CDC released a recent report warning travelers that the virus could leave infectious material in the air[16] they were careful to say that it was not capable of spreading like other airborne viruses such as the common cold or flu.

But, with the way the virus has mutated and spread thus far, to say that the world's top medical professionals and health officials are worried would be an understatement. Ebola has contacted more humans in the last 9 months than all previous outbreaks over the last 40 years combined. The concern, according to officials, is that it has had an opportunity to mutate and it could eventually go airborne.

What is not getting said publicly, despite briefings and discussions in the inner circles of the world's public health agencies, is that we are in totally uncharted waters and that Mother Nature is the only force in charge of the crisis at this time.

There are two possible future chapters to this story that should keep us up at night.

The first possibility is that the Ebola virus spreads from West Africa to megacities in other regions of the developing world. This outbreak is very different from the 19 that have occurred in Africa over the past 40 years. It is much easier to control Ebola infections in isolated villages. But there has been a 300 percent increase in Africa's population over the last four decades, much of it in large city slums. What happens when an infected person yet to become ill travels by plane to Lagos, Nairobi, Kinshasa or Mogadishu — or even Karachi, Jakarta, Mexico City or Dhaka?

The second possibility is one that virologists are loath to discuss openly but are definitely considering in private: **that an Ebola virus could mutate to become transmissible through the air.** You can now get Ebola only through direct contact with bodily fluids. But viruses like Ebola are notoriously sloppy in replicating, meaning the virus entering one person may be genetically different from the virus entering the next.

> *The current Ebola virus's hyper-evolution is unprecedented; there has been more human-to-human transmission in the past four months*

*than most likely occurred in the last 500
to 1,000 years. Each new infection
represents trillions of throws of the
genetic dice.*

*If certain mutations occurred, it would
mean that just breathing would put one
at risk of contracting Ebola.*

Source: New York Times[17]

In the event of the Ebola virus going airborne,
research models show that it would quickly
spread to all corners of the globe, infecting and
killing millions.

U.S. hospitals are already preparing intake
areas[18] in case the virus hits home and a
Congressional report released earlier this year
says that Ebola detection kits and mobile

---

[17] http://www.nytimes.com/2014/09/12/opinion/what-
were-afraid-to-say-about-
ebola.html?emc=edit_tnt_20140911&nlid=745484&tnte
mail0=y&_r=1
[18] http://www.shtfplan.com/headline-news/u-s-
hospitals-prep-for-ebola-outbreak-cases-may-exceed-
100000-by-december-the-numbers-are-really-
scary_09012014

response facilities have been to National Guard units in all fifty states.[19]

Thus, while the public remains oblivious to the seriousness of the threat, the government is rapidly ramping up preparations.

However, it may all be for naught should the current Ebola strains become transmissible by air. In such an event millions will contract the virus and the medical systems in the United States will be overwhelmed. Moreover, any experimental vaccines may be slow in coming due to massive global demand and limited supplies.

This leaves prevention on an individual scale the only viable strategy.

Moreover, should such an event grip the world, millions of people would be in panic mode. Normal systems of commerce would likely break down, leaving many without food, clean water, and power. Thus, preparing for a scenario where the world as we know it literally comes to a screeching halt is also important to consider.

---

[19] http://www.shtfplan.com/headline-news/congressional-report-ebola-bio-kits-deployed-to-national-guard-units-in-all-50-states_07292014

To be clear, Ebola has not yet achieved an airborne mutation in humans that we are aware of (though research has shown that it has been carried by breathing between animals). But, just because it has happened yet, doesn't mean it can't, especially considering the number of official cases reported so far.

In 1918 the Spanish flu killed as many as 50 million people, roughly 5% of the world's population. Can you imagine the implications of an airborne Ebola virus with a mortality rate of 50% to 90%?

How is Ebola transmitted?

The World Health Organization[20] provides the following information regarding the transmission of Ebola.

> *Infection occurs from direct contact through broken skin or mucous membranes with the blood, or other bodily fluids or secretions (stool, urine, saliva, semen) of infected people. Infection can also occur if broken skin or mucous membranes of a healthy person come into contact with environments that have become contaminated with an Ebola patient's infectious fluids such as soiled clothing, bed linen, or used needles.*

> *More than 100 health-care workers have been exposed to the virus while caring for Ebola patients. This happens because they may not have been wearing personal protection equipment or were not properly applying infection prevention and control measures when caring for the patients. Health-care providers*

20

http://www.who.int/mediacentre/factsheets/fs103/en/

at all levels of the health system –
hospitals, clinics, and health posts –
should be briefed on the nature of
the disease and how it is
transmitted, and strictly follow
recommended infection control
precautions.

**WHO does not advise families or
communities to care for individuals
who may present with symptoms of
Ebola virus disease in their homes**.
Rather, seek treatment in a hospital
or treatment centre staffed by
doctors and nurses qualified and
equipped to treat Ebola virus
victims. If you do choose to care for
your loved one at home, WHO
strongly advises you to notify your
local public health authority and
receive appropriate training,
equipment (gloves and personal
protective equipment [PPE]) for
treatment, instructions on proper
removal and disposal of PPE, and
information on how to prevent
further infection and transmission of
the disease to yourself, other family
members, or the community.

Additional transmission has
occurred in communities during

funerals and burial rituals. Burial ceremonies in which mourners have direct contact with the body of the deceased person have played a role in the transmission of Ebola. Persons who have died of Ebola must be handled using strong protective clothing and gloves and must be buried immediately. WHO advises that the deceased be handled and buried by trained case management professionals, who are equipped to properly bury the dead.

People are infectious as long as their blood and secretions contain the virus. For this reason, infected patients receive close monitoring from medical professionals and receive laboratory tests to ensure the virus is no longer circulating in their systems before they return home. When the medical professionals determine it is okay for the patient to return home, they are no longer infectious and cannot infect anyone else in their communities. Men who have recovered from the illness can still spread the virus to their partner through their semen for up to 7 weeks after recovery. For this reason, it is important for men to avoid sexual intercourse for at least 7 weeks after recovery or to wear condoms if having sexual intercourse during 7 weeks after recovery.

Ebola:

How It Kills May Surprise You

By Lisa Egan

As several countries in West Africa continue to struggle with the worst Ebola outbreak in history, the news worldwide has been flooded with stories about the mysterious and horrifying virus.

Photos of victims with the telltale hemorrhagic rash, bleeding from the eyes, ears, and nose, and stories of the stricken vomiting and coughing up blood add to the terror associated with this deadly virus.

But what exactly IS Ebola, and how does it kill?

Ebola is an infection with a virus of the family *Filoviridae*, genus Ebolavirus. So far, only two members of this family of viruses have been identified - Marburgvirus and Ebolavirus. Five subspecies of Ebolavirus have been identified, four of which can cause disease in humans[21]:

---

[21] http://www.cdc.gov/vhf/ebola/about.html

- Ebola virus (Zaire ebolavirus)
- Sudan virus (Sudan ebolavirus)
- Taï Forest virus (Taï Forest ebolavirus, formerly Côte d'Ivoire ebolavirus)
- Bundibugyo virus (Bundibugyo ebolavirus)

The fifth subspecies, Reston virus (Reston ebolavirus), is the one that has not caused disease in humans (but it can be fatal in non-human primates). This is the strain that killed dozens of lab monkeys at a research facility in Reston, VA, in 1989. Four workers at that facility tested positive for Ebola. In 1996, nine lab workers were exposed to this strain after handling infected animals. None of those infected developed symptoms or became ill, but they did develop antibodies to the strain. It is possible that the Reston strain can be transmitted via small-particle aerosols (airborne), but that hasn't been confirmed.

Filovirus infections are transmitted via close personal contact with an infected individual or their bodily fluids (including through contact with contaminated medical equipment).

According to the CDC[22], "although in the laboratory the viruses display some capability of infection through small-particle aerosols,

---

[22] http://www.cdc.gov/vhf/virus-families/filoviridae.html

airborne spread among humans has not been clearly demonstrated."

A study released last week showed that the strain causing the current outbreak in West Africa has gone through a surprisingly high amount of genetic drift. Those mutations may make treatment and diagnosis harder.

But can those mutations make Ebola virus change enough to become truly airborne, like the flu?

In his article "Can Ebola Go Airborne?"[23] Dr. Scott Gottlieb said it is possible, but unlikely:

> The widespread belief is that the Ebola virus would be very unlikely to change in a way that would allow the individual virus particles to be concentrated, and remain suspended in respiratory secretions — and then infect contacts through inhalation. The Ebola virus is comprised of ribonucleic acid (RNA). Such a structure makes it prone to undergoing rapid genetic changes.
>
> But to become airborne, a lot of unlikely events would need to occur.

---

[23] http://www.forbes.com/fdc/welcome_mjx.shtml

Ebola's RNA genome would have to mutate to the point where the coating that surrounds the virus particles (the protein capsid) is no longer susceptible to harsh drying effects of being suspended in air. To be spread through the air, it also generally helps if the virus is concentrated in the lungs of affected patients.

For humans, this is not the case. Ebola generally isn't an infection of the lungs. The main organ that the virus targets is the liver. That is why patients stricken with Ebola develop very high amounts of the virus in the blood and in the feces, and not in their respiratory secretions.

Regarding the chances of an outbreak occurring in the United States, Dr. Gottlieb had this to say:

We will certainly see cases diagnosed here, and perhaps even experience some isolated clusters of disease. Health-care workers in advanced Western nations maintain infection controls that can curtail the spread of non-airborne diseases like Ebola.

The current outbreak in West Africa is caused by the Zaire ebolavirus. If infection is properly diagnosed quickly, and treatment is given promptly, a full recovery is likely.

However, the very nature of the Ebola virus can make early detection tricky. Early symptoms are similar to those of many far less harmless diseases. Fever, headache, weakness, diarrhea, and vomiting often present in the early stages, and can lead to a misdiagnosis - and delayed treatment.

What is intriguing - and terrifying - about Ebola is that the virus itself doesn't kill people - the immune system's reaction to it does.

"The normal job of the immune system is to eliminate infections," virologist Christopher Basler explained to NPR[24]. "But when it's activated at extreme levels or it's out of control, it becomes damaging to the host."

In his article titled Ebola: A Dangerous Virus, But How Does It Really Kill?[25], Professor

---

[24]

http://www.npr.org/blogs/goatsandsoda/2014/08/26/342451672/how-ebola-kills-you-its-not-the-virus
[25] http://saharareporters.com/2014/09/01/ebola-dangerous-virus-how-does-it-really-kill-professor-edward-oparaoji

Edward Oparaoji explains how Ebola invades the body and causes the immune system to go into overdrive:

> It disguises itself and stealthily evades detection and "arrest" by the "security guard" - dendritic cells and macrophages. Once inside and secured, the virus disarms the "security guard" rendering them incapable of sending signals for help to the protective "commandoes" - the antibodies and cytokines, to eliminate the "suspect" Ebola. As a result, the virus starts to multiply and invade more cells with reckless abandon, unchallenged, causing cells to die and explode. It is at this stage that the (host) immune system suddenly becomes aware that it has been overrun.

He goes on to explain how the immune system responds:

> It then begins a belated over the top uncoordinated defense, launching its entire immunological arsenal at once, through massive release of cytokines - the (host) immune system equivalence of "shock and awe" response to the

already widely spread virus. This most extreme immune response, which also signals the terminal phase of the infection, is referred to as the "cytokine storm"- It is this cytokine storm, the host response to the Ebola that kills. During this condition, the (host) immune system turns on itself, attacking every organ in the body, bursting blood vessels and making the infected person bleed both internally and externally, through the orifices (eyes, nose, etc.). This also involves vomits and diarrhea, causing severe low blood pressure and/or hypotensive shock and subsequently, death.

Other viral infections like Bird Flu and SARS can cause the immune system to launch an intense attack as well, but not with as much ferocity as it does with Ebola.

Survival requires stopping the cytokine storm and resulting hypotensive shock from occurring. Professor Oparaoji explains how this is done:

This can be accomplished through appropriate timely Anti-Ebola drug (ZMapp) or vaccine treatment, when available, and/or aggressive effective supportive treatment - such as maintenance of oxygenation, fluid and electrolyte therapy, blood pressure control with vasopressors, prevention and treatment of secondary infections, pain control and nutritional support, among others.

He also points out that treatment with the ZMAPP drug and Nigeria's supportive treatment protocol don't yield results that are that much different: 33% of people treated with ZMAPP have died, compared to 40% who were treated per Nigeria's standard supportive treatment.

Medical missionaries Dr. Kent Brantly and Nancy Writebol were the first people to use ZMAPP. Both received supportive care at Emory University Hospital in Atlanta, and both have fully recovered. Dr. Brantly also received a unit of donated blood from a 14-year-old boy who recovered from Ebola. Similar treatment (via plasma antibodies) was used in an outbreak in 1995, with stunning results: 7 of the 8 treated with blood from convalesced patients survived.[26]

---

[26] http://www.newsweek.com/20-year-old-ebola-treatment-could-save-kent-brantly-262552

But was their recovery due to the use of ZMAPP or something else?

At this point, we don't know:

> "They are the very first individuals to have ever receive this agent," Dr. Bruce Ribner, director of Emory's Infectious Disease Unit, told a news conference.[27] "There is no prior experience with it, and frankly, we do not know whether it helped them, whether it made no difference, or even, theoretically, if it delayed their recovery."

Doctors who have experience treating Ebola say that early and aggressive supportive care (like the care Professor Oparaoji described) is crucial to recovery. The physical condition of a person infected with Ebola also matters:

> "And clearly for any acutely ill patient, nutritional status is extremely important," Ribner said. "If you have somebody who's well-nourished and somebody who is poorly nourished and they suffer the same illness, infectious

---

[27] http://www.nbcnews.com/storyline/ebola-virus-outbreak/what-cured-ebola-patients-kent-brantly-nancy-writebol-n186131

*or otherwise, the person with better
nutrition has better survival outlook."*

ZMAPP is one of several Ebola treatments being developed. But, no matter which drug - if any - proves to be a useful treatment, time will be of the essence. It only takes viruses a few days to replicate and spread, and once the damage becomes widespread it can be impossible to reverse.

Regarding treatment with the blood of convalesced patients, well, it has been said that it would take a lot of plasma to make that a viable option. At this point, it doesn't appear that anyone is seriously pursuing the use of that treatment modality, although there has been some discussion[28] about it.

As with any disease, an ounce of prevention is worth a pound of cure.

Part Two:

---

[28] http://www.bloomberg.com/news/2014-08-18/blood-of-ebola-survivors-holds-therapy-potential-for-sick.html

How You Can Protect Your Family from Ebola

Prepping for an Ebola Lockdown: No one goes out, no one comes in

By Daisy Luther

Are you prepared to go into lockdown mode if the Ebola virus begins to spread across the country?

Hopefully, fears of a possible Ebola pandemic are exaggerated and being fanned by a government with an agenda[29] and greedy pharmaceutical companies[30].

However...

Six people fell ill in New York City and are being tested for the virus. Paul Joseph Watson of Prison Planet wrote[31]:

> "In an apparent attempt to avoid hysteria, U.S. health authorities are

---

[29] http://www.thedailysheeple.com/what-are-the-odds-nyc-tests-patient-for-ebola-just-days-after-largest-bio-attack-drill-in-city-history_082014
[30] http://www.thedailysheeple.com/doctor-theres-not-enough-panic-and-customers-to-make-an-ebola-vaccine-oh-really_082014
[31] http://www.prisonplanet.com/u-s-health-authorities-concealing-number-of-suspected-ebola-victims-from-public.html

withholding details about a number of suspected Ebola victims from the public."

With something that displays itself as gruesomely as Ebola, with seizures and uncontrollable bleeding from every orifice, it's unrealistic to think that a cover-up can last long. If this continues to spread, there's no way that the government can keep it under wraps. In a place as populated as NYC, there's no telling how many people the possible victims have come into contact with. This is NOT going to be easy to contain. The virus is spreading far more rapidly than it has in the past in West Africa[32], giving some people reason to believe it has mutated into something more easily transmissible.

This reminds me of that scene in the movie *Contagion*, where the CDC experts have their quiet, closed-door meetings and discuss preventing a panic. (If you haven't seen that movie lately, I suggest you watch it, perhaps with your older children, to open the discussion of how pandemics can spread rapidly.) In the movie, the officials seem

---

[32] http://www.thedailysheeple.com/the-bizarre-growth-of-the-ebola-outbreak-this-graph-says-it-all_082014

almost more intent on keeping it quiet than they do on stopping the spread of the illness.

There are a lot of facts that are being kept quiet[33]. The government seems really excited about producing an untested vaccine and jabbing us all with it[34]. Because of this insistence on secrecy and the fact that you just can't trust the government, you may not have a lot of warning before things get really bad. Consider *this* your warning. You need to be prepared to go into family lockdown mode for at least six weeks. Incidentally, this begs the question of why our government has not gone into a similar lockdown mode, instead of opening the floodgates for illegal immigrants and tourists from other countries during a global health crisis.

How do you know when it's time to go into lockdown?

Avoiding contact with people who have the illness is the only way to prevent getting it.

---

[33] http://theeconomiccollapseblog.com/archives/25-critical-facts-about-this-ebola-outbreak-that-every-american-needs-to-know
[34] http://sgtreport.com/2014/08/contagion-and-the-u-s-governments-ebola-vaccine/

Isolating yourselves is the best way to stay safe and healthy.

This is the tricky part: How do you know that the time has come to get the family inside and lock the doors behind you? Lizzie Bennett, a retired medical professional, wrote[35] some of the most blunt, honest things you will read from a person who worked in this field. Bennett recommends social distancing as the *only* effective way to protect yourself and your family from an outbreak of disease. (**Editor's note**: *Lizzie's article, in its entirety, follows this one*)

> *How long you should remain isolated depends primarily on where you live. For those in towns and cities it will be for much longer than those living in rural retreats where human contact is minimal. Though those fortunate enough to live in such surroundings should remember that if the situation is dire enough, people will leave the cities looking for safety in less populated areas. In large centres of population there will be more people moving around, legally or otherwise, each of these individuals represents a possible uptick in the disease rates, allowing the*

---

[35] http://undergroundmedic.com/?p=74

*spread to continue longer than it would
have they stayed indoors and/or out of
circulation. Even when the initial phase
is on the wane, or has passed through
an area, people travelling into that area
can bring it back with them triggering a
second wave of disease as people are
now emerging from their isolation...*

...

*One hundred miles is my buffer zone for
disease, of course it could already be in
my city, but practicalities dictate that I
will not stay away from people because
hundreds in Europe are dropping like
flies. Maps of disease spread look like a
locust swarm moving across the
country and this allows disease spread
to be tracked on an hour by hour basis.
One of the few instances where
mainstream media will be useful.*

Once you've gone into lockdown, how long
you must stay there is dependent on the
spread of the illness. Times will vary. Bennett
suggests these guidelines:

Once the doors were locked we would stay
there for at least two weeks after the last case
within 100 miles is reported. A government all
clear would be weighed against how long it

had been since the last case was reported in the area I have designated as my buffer zone. There is of course still the chance that someone from outside the area will bring the disease in with them causing a second wave of illness. You cannot seal off cities to prevent this. Going out after self-imposed isolation should be kept to a minimum for as long as possible, and if you don't have to, then don't do it. Far better to let those that are comfortable being out and about get on with it and see if any new cases emerge before exposing yourself and your family to that possibility.

What does it mean to go into lockdown?

This Ebola thing could go bad in a hurry. And by bad I mean that it has killed well over half of the people who've contracted it in West Africa. Not only do we have the possibility of Ebola to contend with, but several varieties of plague are also on the uptick over the past couple of months, something that has been put on the back burner due to the fear of Ebola. A city in China was locked down last week due to the Bubonic Plague[36] and the Black Plague caused one man to die and 3

---

[36] http://mashable.com/2014/07/22/chinese-town-on-lock-down-after-bubonic-plague-death/

more people to become ill in Colorado[37] last month.

If the situation hits close enough to home that you decide to go it's time to isolate yourselves, the rules to this are intractable.

No one goes out. No one comes in.

I know this sounds harsh, but there are to be no exceptions. If you make exceptions, you might as well go wrestle with runny-nosed strangers at the local Wal-Mart and then come home and hug your children, because it's the same thing.

Once you have gone into lockdown mode, it means that the supplies you have on hand are the supplies you have to see you through. You can't run out to the store and get something you've forgotten.

That means if a family member shows up, they have to go into quarantine for at least 4 weeks, during which time they are not allowed access to the home or family, nor are they allowed to go out in public. Set up an area on your property that is far from your home for them to hang out for their month of quarantine. If at

---

[37] http://www.bloomberg.com/news/2014-07-18/four-cases-of-life-threatening-plague-found-in-colorado.html

the end of the month they are presenting no symptoms, then they can come in.

It sadly means that you may be forced to turn someone away if they are ill, because to help them means to risk your family.

Now is the time to plan with your preparedness group how you intend to handle the situation. Will you shelter together, in the same location, and reserve a secondary location to retreat to if the situation worsens further or if someone becomes ill? Will you shelter separately because of the nature of the emergency? Decide together on what event and proximity will trigger you to go into lockdown mode. Make your plan and stick to it, regardless of pressure from those who think you are over-reacting, the school that your children have stopped attending, and any other external influences. If you've decided that there is a great enough risk that you need to go into lockdown, you must adhere to your plan.

Social Distancing as a Means to Avoid Contagion

By Lizzie Bennett

Ebola is on most people's minds at the moment, more so since the United States and Germany took the decision to fly Ebola patients from West Africa to hospitals in Atlanta and Hamburg.

Ebola Zaire is one of five strains of Ebola that are currently known, only one, Ebola Reston is not fatal in humans. Ebola Zaire, the strain currently in circulation has a death rate approaching 90%.

During pandemics or epidemics, which are localized disease outbreaks, our not so esteemed leaders will most likely start by issuing advisories to avoid large gatherings of people, baseball games, football matches that sort of thing. The next step is closures of such venues, games will be cancelled to limit the spread of the disease. One up from this is the closure of large institutions, such as college campuses. This is followed by the temporary closure of schools, and other public buildings such as council offices, job centers and libraries, and finally, cinemas and even churches may be closed. Airlines may cancel flights or flights into and out of affected areas may be banned by government order to contain an outbreak.

The final imposed restriction is curfew. Individuals will not be allowed to move around freely in order to limit the spread of the disease. This decision will not be taken lightly by governments...unless they are thinking Agenda 21 and seize the chance to reduce the population by a few million. Enforced curfew means that many of those who have not prepared are going to die, either of dehydration and starvation, or by bullet when they break the curfew in their hunt for supplies. In view of the estimated amounts of unprepared people out there, security forces would in my opinion, be so overwhelmed by the numbers of those breaking the curfew they would not have the option of rounding them up, many will die.

As an individual, you may have already decided not to send your child to school, you may have already driven across the state or even the country to get an older child home from college. You are, if you are reading this, probably well stocked and good to go if you decide to stay away from everyone until the situation improves. How long do you need to stay holed up for? When will it be safe to leave your home? What precautions do you take on returning if you really have to go out?

There can be no rule of thumb for how long you need to stay isolated for, but if any of you think a month will do it you need to think again. Although diseases spread at different rates, have different incubation times and are infectious at different times during their course they all rely on one thing. A supply of suitable hosts.

The supply of hosts, in this case us, is known as the herd, and providing the herd is big enough the disease will keep spreading. If the herd is too small, the disease will die out, this is the basis of shutting down sporting fixtures and campuses, reducing the size of the herd.

Microbiologists, as a baseline figure will make an assumption based on how a disease has spread in the past. For example, that one infected person will go on to infect 20 others. Some diseases such as Hansen's disease (leprosy) although contagious, has a much lower infection rate than this, other diseases such as pandemic influenza, are much higher. 20 is considered a mean average with a virulent flu strain. So one teacher can infect 20 kids. Each of those 20 kids can infect 20 more people: that makes 400. Each of those 400 can infect 20 people: that makes 8000. Disease spreads very quickly, and if you have something with a short incubation period, you have thousands of infected people around at the same time. The problem is, so many of the worst diseases start off resembling the common cold, fever, aches, sore throat, and headache. If presenting during the winter 'flu season' it can go un-noticed for even longer. By the time it is realized it is more than just a regular bug doing the rounds the situation is well on its way to being out of control, it will keep spreading as long as there is people for it to spread to.

How long you should remain isolated depends primarily on where you live. For those in towns and cities it will be for much longer than those living in rural retreats where human contact is minimal. Though those fortunate enough to live in such surroundings should remember that if the situation is dire enough, people will leave the cities looking for safety in less populated areas. In large centers of population there will be more people moving around, legally or otherwise, each of these individuals represents a possible uptick in the disease rates, allowing the spread to continue longer than it would have they stayed indoors and/or out of circulation. Even when the initial phase is on the wane, or has passed through an area, people travelling into that area can bring it back with them triggering a second wave of disease as people are now emerging from their isolation.

On finding out there may be a major event in the offing, that people were becoming sickened I would dissect the information I had and find out as much as I could about the condition. This would not take more than an hour or two.

On finding it is a definite threat I would go shopping....make sure that any holes in my preps are, as far as I am able, filled. I would be looking for the usual, easy cook long life foods and bottled water, lots of bottled water. If systems break down due to staff sickness or death other diseases may spring up and so many are waterborne I would store as much as I could. Waste collections may be affected, thick rubbish bags, and several more gallons of bleach to keep the outside areas of the home free from pathogens delivered by rats etc. who will be attracted by mountains of garbage would be a priority.

Lots of pairs of disposable decorator's coveralls, disposable gloves and a filtered face masks would be next. If I had to go out these would be discarded before re-entering my home.

Fly spray or fly papers should be on every preppers list, but most of us severely underestimate the amount we will need. Any crisis that causes rubbish to build will see a massive increase in their numbers, they are also effective germ carriers and spreaders and should be viewed as a threat to your general good health. Although they may not be capable of carrying the disease that is causing the crisis secondary illnesses often occur in such situations.

The idea of shopping at this point is to preserve my stored preps for the maximum amount of time. Pandemics and diseases go in waves, often returning several times before the crisis is finally over. After the first wave has passed, there is no guarantee that life will operate as it did before. Depending on the mortality rate of the disease the population may have thinned considerably, the food chain could well be affected and municipal services may well have stopped or be severely reduced. The last minute shopping trip could well be the last time you are able to supply yourself with what you need.

I would continue these trips, gathering as many extra supplies as I could until I heard of the first case within one hundred miles of my home. At that point self-imposed isolation comes into effect. One hundred miles is my buffer zone for disease, of course it could already be in my city, but practicalities dictate that I will not stay away from people because hundreds in Europe are dropping like flies. Maps of disease spread look like a locust swarm moving across the country and this allows disease spread to be tracked on an hour by hour basis. One of the few instances where mainstream media will be useful.

Once the doors were locked we would stay there for at least two weeks after the last case within 100 miles is reported. A government all clear would be weighed against how long it had been since the last case was reported in the area I have designated as my buffer zone. There is of course still the chance that someone from outside the area will bring the disease in with them causing a second wave of illness. You cannot seal off cities to prevent this. Going out after self-imposed isolation should be kept to a minimum for as long as possible, and if you don't have to, then don't do it. Far better to let those that are comfortable being out and about get on with it and see if any new cases emerge before exposing yourself and your family to that possibility.

As with most things we prepare for there is and will continue to be massive uncertainty during times of crisis. Diseases can be unpredictable and are capable of mutating at an alarming rate. New emerging diseases, and re-emerging diseases are often zoonoses, that is diseases that jump the species barrier from animal to human and these unfortunately can be the most unpredictable of all.

The continental United States has seen unprecedented heat in many areas of late, drought conditions prevail in many areas. Animals will migrate in search of water, as humans have done for millennia. Bubonic plague is present in many animals in the Sierra Nevada area, Hantavirus greatly favors dry conditions. West Nile virus and other mosquito spread disease is on the increase. Last winter the UK saw numerous floods, rodents are on the march, looking for drier, higher ground. They bring with them a massively increased risk of leptospirosis. Cholera is now not only a problem in Haiti, but in Cuba, having reached Havana earlier this week. Cuba to the closest point of Key West is 90.5 miles...inside my buffer zone limit though admittedly the ocean makes spread less likely than if they were joined by land and the cholera is not yet epidemic let alone pandemic.

Pandemics have occurred before and they will happen again. Localized epidemics are quite common. A little thought as to how you would deal with not only the contagion but the other issues that could arise from it may well save you a great deal of grief in the long term. No crisis remains isolated. Each and every one of them will have a knock on effect. You may survive the pandemic, but what about the three months' worth of rubbish in the streets, the plague of rats and the thousands of unburied bodies left in its wake?

Think ahead and have a plan, and as I have learned from so many preppers, have a backup plan.

Prepare for the Possibility of Illness in your Family

By Daisy Luther

During an Ebola outbreak, every minor pain, sniffle or fever will be greeted with immediate diagnostic fervor worthy of an episode of the TV medical drama, *House*. Before succumbing to panic, it's vital that you be familiar with the symptoms of the disease.

The CDC offers this information[38] on the symptoms of the dreaded Ebola hemorrhagic fever, now renamed Ebola virus disease

- *Fever (greater than 38.6°C or 101.5°F)*
- *Severe headache*
- *Muscle pain*
- *Diarrhea*
- *Vomiting*
- *Abdominal (stomach) pain*

Symptoms may appear anywhere from 2 to 21 days after exposure to ebolavirus, although 8-10 days is most common.

---

[38] http://www.cdc.gov/vhf/ebola/symptoms/

The World Health Organization fact sheet[39] says:

> EVD is a severe acute viral illness often characterized by the sudden onset of fever, intense weakness, muscle pain, headache and sore throat. This is followed by vomiting, diarrhoea, rash, impaired kidney and liver function, and in some cases, both internal and external bleeding. Laboratory findings include low white blood cell and platelet counts and elevated liver enzymes.
>
> People are infectious as long as their blood and secretions contain the virus. Ebola virus was isolated from semen 61 days after onset of illness in a man who was infected in a laboratory.
>
> The incubation period, that is, the time interval from infection with the virus to onset of symptoms, is 2 to 21 days.

39
http://www.who.int/mediacentre/factsheets/fs103/en/

Diagnosis

Other diseases that should be ruled out before a diagnosis of EVD can be made include: malaria, typhoid fever, shigellosis, cholera, leptospirosis, plague, rickettsiosis, relapsing fever, meningitis, hepatitis and other viral haemorrhagic fevers.

Ebola virus infections can be diagnosed definitively in a laboratory through several types of tests:

- *antibody-capture enzyme-linked immunosorbent assay (ELISA)*
- *antigen detection tests*
- *serum neutralization test*
- *reverse transcriptase polymerase chain reaction (RT-PCR) assay*
- *electron microscopy*
- *virus isolation by cell culture.*

Samples from patients are an extreme biohazard risk; testing should be conducted under maximum biological containment conditions.
Vaccine and treatment

No licensed vaccine for EVD is available. Several vaccines are being tested, but none are available for clinical use.

Severely ill patients require intensive supportive care. Patients are frequently dehydrated and require oral rehydration with solutions containing electrolytes or intravenous fluids.

No specific treatment is available. New drug therapies are being evaluated.

In the event that a member of your group becomes ill, they need to immediately be quarantined from the rest of the group. By the time they're showing symptoms, it could be too late to prevent the spread of illness but effort should still be taken to isolate them.

Here are some tips on isolating a patient.

- The sick room should be sealed off from the rest of the house. Use a heavy tarp over the doorway to the room on the inside and the outside. This will make a small breezeway for the caretaker to go in and out.

- The caretaker should cover up with disposable clothing, gloves, shoe covers, and hair covers.
- The caretaker should wear an N95 mask.
- The caretaker should "decontaminate" immediately upon leaving the sick room, by stripping off all exposed clothing and either discarding it or putting it in the washing machine, on hot, with bleach. Then the caretaker should immediately shower completely, including the washing of hair. At the absolute minimum, use soap and water on hands, followed by an alcohol based hand rub.
- The sick person should use disposable dishes and cutlery. All garbage from the sick room should be placed in a heavy garbage bag and burned outdoors immediately.
- The sick person should not leave the room. If there is not a bedroom with a connected bathroom, a bathroom setup should be created within the room. Great care must be taken with the disposal of this waste.

If, heaven forbid, a member of your group succumbs to Ebola, great care must be taken with the disposal of the body. Ebola is contagious even after death. The CDC offers this advice. [40]

> These recommendations give guidance on the safe handling of human remains that may contain Ebola virus and are for use by personnel who perform postmortem care in U.S. hospitals and mortuaries. In patients who die of Ebola virus infection, virus can be detected throughout the body. Ebola virus can be transmitted in postmortem care settings by laceration and puncture with contaminated instruments used during postmortem care, through direct handling of human remains without appropriate personal protective equipment, and through splashes of blood or other body fluids (e.g. urine, saliva, feces) to unprotected mucosa (e.g., eyes, nose, or mouth) which occur during postmortem care.

40
http://www.cdc.gov/vhf/ebola/hcp/guidance-safe-handling-human-remains-ebola-patients-us-hospitals-mortuaries.html

- *Only personnel trained in handling infected human remains, and wearing PPE, should touch, or move, any Ebola-infected remains.*
- *Handling of human remains should be kept to a minimum.*
- *Autopsies on patients who die of Ebola should be **avoided.** If an autopsy is necessary, the state health department and CDC should be consulted regarding additional precautions.*

Definitions for Terms Used in this Guidance

Cremation: The act of reducing human remains to ash by intense heat.

Hermetically sealed casket: A casket that is airtight and secured against the escape of microorganisms. A casket will be considered hermetically sealed if accompanied by valid documentation that it has been hermetically sealed AND, on visual inspection, the seal appears not to have been broken.

Leakproof bag: A body bag that is puncture-resistant and sealed in a manner so as to contain all contents and prevent leakage of fluids during handling, transport, or shipping.

Personal protective equipment for postmortem care personnel

- **Personal protective equipment (PPE)**: *Prior to contact with body, postmortem care personnel must wear PPE consisting of: surgical scrub suit, surgical cap, impervious gown with full sleeve coverage, eye protection (e.g., face shield, goggles), facemask, shoe covers, and double surgical gloves. Additional PPE (leg coverings, apron) might be required in certain situations (e.g., copious amounts of blood, vomit, feces, or other body fluids that can contaminate the environment).*

- **Putting on, wearing, removing, and disposing of protective equipment**: *PPE should be in place **BEFORE** contact with the body, worn during the process of* collection and placement in body bags, and should be removed immediately after and discarded as regulated medical waste. Use caution when removing PPE as to avoid contaminating the wearer. Hand hygiene (washing your hands thoroughly with soap and water or an alcohol based hand rub) should be performed immediately following the removal of PPE. If hands are visibly soiled, use soap and water.

Postmortem preparation

- **Preparation of the body**: At the site of death, the body should be wrapped in a plastic shroud. Wrapping of the body should be done in a way that prevents contamination of the outside of the shroud. Change your gown or gloves if they become heavily contaminated with blood or body fluids. Leave any intravenous lines or endotracheal tubes that may be present in place. Avoid washing or cleaning the body. After wrapping, the body should be immediately placed in a leak-proof plastic bag not less than 150 μm thick and zippered closed The bagged body should then be placed in another leak-proof plastic bag not less than 150 μm thick and zippered closed before being transported to the morgue.

- **Surface decontamination**: Prior to transport to the morgue, perform surface decontamination of the corpse-containing body bags by removing visible soil on outer bag surfaces with EPA-registered disinfectants which can kill a wide range of viruses. Follow the product's label instructions. the visible soil has been removed, reapply the disinfectant to the entire bag surface and allow to air dry. Following the removal of the body, the patient room should be cleaned and disinfected. Reusable equipment should be cleaned and disinfected according to standard procedures. For more information on environmental infection control, please refer to "Interim Guidance _for Environmental Infection Control in_ _Hospitals for Ebola Virus"_ _(http://www.cdc.gov/vhf/ebola/hcp/envir_ _onmental-infection-control-in-_ _hospitals.html)._

- **_Individuals driving or riding in a vehicle carrying human remains:_** _PPE is not required for individuals driving or riding in a vehicle carrying human remains, provided that drivers or riders will not be handling the remains of a suspected or confirmed case of Ebola, and the remains are safely contained and the body bag is disinfected as described above._

Mortuary Care

- _Do not perform embalming. The risks of occupational exposure to Ebola virus while embalming outweighs its advantages; therefore, bodies infected with Ebola virus should not be embalmed._
- _Do not open the body bags._

- *Do not remove remains from the body bags. Bagged bodies should be placed directly into a hermetically sealed casket.*
- *Mortuary care personnel should wear PPE listed above (surgical scrub suit, surgical cap, impervious gown with full sleeve coverage, eye protection (e.g., face shield, goggles), facemask, shoe covers, and double surgical gloves) when handling the bagged remains.*
- *In the event of leakage of fluids from the body bag, thoroughly clean and decontaminate areas of the environment with EPA-registered disinfectants which can kill a broad range of viruses in accordance with label instructions. Reusable equipment should be cleaned and disinfected according to standard procedures. For more information on environmental infection control, please refer to "Interim Guidance for Environmental Infection Control in Hospitals for Ebola Virus" (http://www.cdc.gov/vhf/ebola/hcp/envir*

onmental-infection-control-in-hospitals.html).

Disposition of Remains

- *Remains should be cremated or buried promptly in a hermetically sealed casket.*
- *Once the bagged body is placed in the sealed casket, no additional cleaning is needed unless leakage has occurred.*
- *No PPE is needed when handling the cremated remains or the hermetically sealed closed casket.*

Transportation of human remains

- *Transportation of remains that contain Ebola virus should be minimized to the extent possible.*
- *All transportation, including local transport, for example, for mortuary care or burial, should be coordinated with relevant local and state authorities in advance.*

- *Interstate transport should be coordinated with CDC by calling the Emergency Operations Center at 770-488-7100. The mode of transportation (i.e., airline or ground transport), must be considered carefully, taking into account distance and the most expeditious route. If shipping by air is needed, the remains must be labeled as dangerous goods in accordance with Department of Transportation regulations (49 Code of Federal Regulations 173.196).*
- *Transportation of remains that contain Ebola virus outside the United States would need to comply with the regulations of the country of destination, and should be coordinated in advance with relevant authorities.*

Dealing With Ebola Infected Corpses

By Lizzie Bennett

Many people who have succumbed to Ebola have contracted the disease from handling and disposal of the corpses of loved ones. There is much information out there of how to avoid catching Ebola, setting up a sick room etc., but there is little mention of disposal of infected corpses.

In a national crisis expert teams will be dispatched to collect corpses, but if they are overwhelmed the corpse needs to be dealt with before more infection occurs. In a really extreme situation help may not be forthcoming, and that's what this article is about.

Some may find the following upsetting and rather dispassionate, and for that I'm sorry, but this article isn't about feelings and grieving, it's about staying alive.

Okay, so, a loved one has died of Ebola and you are left with a highly infective corpse. What do you do? Well, first you need to understand what often happens at the time of a 'normal' death, and what always happens at the time of an Ebola death.

Once death occurs degradation starts almost immediately and for bodies not taken away and dealt with by undertakers, morticians and coroners visible signs of decay can start in as little as 15 minutes after death if the conditions are warm and humid.

At the point of death the body starts to cool, within four hours the body will be at or close to the temperature of its surroundings. During this time the skin will have paled visibly and will be waxy looking. Postural lividity caused by blood pooling and coagulating in the lowest part of the body will have occurred so, someone lying face down will be discolored, looking a purple/dark blue color on the front of their body.

The muscles that control the bowel and the bladder will have lost their tonicity, they will be relaxed and moving the body will cause both to evacuate. Rigor Mortis, which literally translates as 'stiffness in death' will be complete at around the 12 hour point after death. The only way to change the position of the body once it has set in is to 'crack' the rigor, literally snapping the muscles to alter the position. Rigor will wear off over the next 18-24 hours but by then, if left the internal organs of the body have started to decay. Gases build up in the gut and intestines and are not passed out of the body as they were in life and this gives the corpse a swollen and bloated appearance.

These gases cause the purification of the internal organs, turning them first to jelly and then to liquid which will escape from the body via the orifices. This foul smelling liquid will exit via the bowels, bladder, mouth, ears, nose and even the eyes.

With a death from Ebola this liquidation of the internal organs has already happened and there WILL be considerable expulsion of these liquids from the body. ALL of those fluids are full of Ebola virus and are highly infective.

If you are nursing someone with Ebola it is a sensible precaution to consider the possibility of their death and limit the exposure of the rest of the family to the disease. A thick plastic sheet or mattress cover should be on the bed, under the sheets of anyone suffering from a contagious disease and this is even more important with Ebola. The reason for this is two-fold.

1. To protect the bed from infection

2. To have a large sheet of plastic in situ already to aid with wrapping the corpse after death

On top of this plastic put a thin sheet, and then another layer of plastic such as a decorator's sheet and then make up the bed as you normally would.

As I explained above there will be a good deal of infectious bodily fluids expelled at the point of, or just after death. Leave them where they are, make no attempt to clean the deceased.

Protective gear, which you should have been wearing to nurse the patient anyway should be reinforced. Put on another pair of gloves, then another coverall, and then a third pair of gloves over the cuffs of the coverall. This is important because it effectively gives you multi-layer protection from secretions. Put on overshoes to protect your feet. Rubber boots are better but the coverall needs to go on after the boots to prevent anything getting inside them.

Okay, moving on:

1. Carefully un-tuck the bedding to the level of the uppermost plastic sheet. Bring it across the deceased, do not

tuck it under them as the risk of a breech in your clothing is too great.

2. Do not stretch over them, move to the other side of the bed and throw the bedding from that side across, then return to the other side of the bed and pull it down snug, using duct tape fix in place as best you can.

3. Take a strong garbage bag and gather it up as you would when putting on a pair of long socks. Slip it over the feet of the deceased and slide it up the corpse, unfurling as you do so.

4. Take a second bag and repeat working from the head down.

5. Duct tape the bags together on the top of the body, do not force your hands and arms underneath.

6. Un-tuck the lower plastic sheet and wrap from the sides first. Tape in place.

7. Repeat the garbage bag procedure but this time when they are securely taped roll the deceased to one side TOWARDS YOU and tape where you can see, at the back. Move to the other side of the bed, roll the deceased TOWARDS YOU and apply more tape. The reason for doing this is to prevent the deceased falling off the bed which could displace the wrappings and contaminate both you and the room.

8. Roll up a light colored sheet leaving about two feet unrolled and lay it along the length of the deceased. The unrolled portion should hang over the side of the bed. Move to the other side of the bed and roll the deceased towards you. Tuck the rolled portion of the sheet under the corpse and gently lay the deceased back down.

9. Go to the other side of the bed, where the sheet is hanging over the edge of the bed and roll the deceased towards you. You will see the rolled sheet in the center of the bed. Push it away from you, it will unroll over to the other edge of the bed. Lay the deceased back down.

10. You now have a wrapped body lying on a white sheet. Pull the sheet down over the head and tape in place. Repeat with the foot end and then the sides, securing each portion of the sheet in place before moving on. The light colored sheet will show you if there is any seepage, a final "warning light" for want of a better term.

The body is now ready to be moved. At least two people should do this to avoid damaging the protective wrapping. Where possible Ebola patients should be nursed on the ground floor of a home to facilitate easier body removal should the need arise.

Ebola victims may be buried, but burials should be in an isolated area where there is no possibility of any run off caused by rain or flooding damaging the wrapping of the body and the remains ending up in water courses. Graves should be very deep to discourage animal disturbance of the remains which could result in the spread of the disease.

Unless you are in a rural location cremation may be the best option. It's unlikely that a body will fully cremate outside of a crematorium so everything possible should be done to ensure complete disposal.

In order to cremate a body you need high heat and good airflow for a considerable amount of time. To achieve this there will ideally be some kind of platform for the bodies to rest on with the fire built underneath this, and then combustible material placed on and around the bodies. If a reusable platform can be built all the better. Piles of bricks or rubble crisscrossed with metal posts or beams, or a metal bed frame would be one way of saving precious fuel, a pyre for multiple bodies is going to take a great deal of it. Regardless of how you construct your pyre the bodies need to be well off the ground or they will not combust effectively, there has to be good airflow all around to get anywhere near complete combustion.

Open cremation is still practiced in many cultures. It is far less labor intensive and has the advantage that germs and disease are destroyed, but as people across the world who have used fire to destroy evidence of crimes have found, bodies do not burn that well. You may need to add an accelerant at certain points during the cremation to make sure that nothing survives the fire.

A Dakota fire pit, is much more labor intensive that an open cremation but uses far less fuel and due to its construction burns much hotter than an open pyre.

The pit should be at least a foot bigger than the body all around and there should be four air vents around it, one each side, one at the head end and one at the foot. Non-combustible materials should be placed at the bottom of the pit and the fire built on top of this, and the body placed on top of the combustible material used to make the fire.

Whichever method you use stand down wind. The smell of burning flesh is not pleasant and there can be particulate matter in the air that is harmful. Bodies that are cremated move and contract, giving them what pathologists call 'the pugilistic pose' the legs bend at the knees and the arms come up, fists clenches as if taking up a boxing stance. This is normal, but is often accompanied by popping sounds as the muscles contract in the heat. Depending on the amount of gases built up in the bodies there is a risk that some may explode, the same with skulls that are exposed to extreme heat.

Your protective gear should remain in place at this point, until you are certain that the fire is burning well and that you will no longer have to touch the body or its wrappings, or until the body is buried and the soil replaced.

At this point you should wash your gloved hands in a bucket of strong bleach water. Remove the gloves and drop them into an open garbage bag. Then:

1. Before removing the second pair of gloves wash your hands in the bleached water, unzip the coverall and step out of it, drop it in the bag with the first pair of gloves. Remove the overshoes and dispose of them if you are wearing them.
2. Wash your hands in the bleach water and remove the second pair of gloves. They go into the bag.

3. You should now be wearing a mask with a visor, glasses or safety goggles and one pair of gloves, and if you opted for them, rubber boots.
4. If the facemask is tied at the back get someone to cut the tie and remove the mask from your face in one fluid movement. Hold each side and pull it away from you, drop it in the bag. Safety goggles and/or glasses can be dropped into the bucket of bleached water.
5. Still wearing your last pair of gloves remove your shoes, one at a time and slip on clean ones. Put the shoes in the garbage. If you are wearing rubber boots leave them on for a few more minutes.
6. Wash your gloved hands in the bleached water. Remove the gloves and put into the bag.
7. If you are wearing rubber boots getting them off without contaminating yourself can be tricky. One foot at a time stand in the bucket or bowl of bleach. Each foot should be in there for a few minutes. As you remove your foot from the bleach put it directly into a rolled down trash bag. Repeat with the other foot.
8. Final bit of disrobing now. Leaving the trash bag in situ pull off one boot and

put your foot directly into a clean shoe. Repeat with the other foot.

9. The boots should be left in the bags until you can stand them in something and using a strong bleach solution saturate them inside and out before leaving them to dry naturally. Many hospitals have rubber boots that are brightly colored to mark them as those to be used specifically for infected cases...I have a bright purple pair tucked away at home so I know at a glance which boots are which.

10. As soon as possible you should shower, not bathe, take care not to swallow any of the water that rolls down off your hair and keep your eyes closed until you have rinsed the shampoo off.

If Ebola does make it out of Africa all precautions need to be taken to prevent its spread. Having said that there will be deaths, we all know this. Hopefully the authorities will not be overwhelmed but if they are the steps outlined above will massively reduce your chances of contracting the disease from handling a dead body.

The Well-Stocked Sick Room
By Tess Pennington

To decrease the chances of an infectious illness spreading and infecting other household members, it is important that every effort be made to keep the illness in a contained area. Having a sick room in the home can achieve this, as well as assist in limiting the number of people who have close contact with the sick person.

Characteristics of the Ideal Sick Room

To ensure that the sickness is as contained as possible, set up the sick room in a bedroom or another separate room in the house. Ensure that the room has good lighting, a window that opens, and easy access to a personal bathroom with a sink and running water.

Prevention is Key

To avoid other family members falling ill, try to limit the exposure of the sick person to the other family members. This includes making sure that any communal areas (kitchen, bathroom, etc.) be thoroughly cleaned with disinfectant each day to avoid the transmission of germs. Towels, water bottles, drinking glasses, and other personal care items used by the sick person, should not be used by other family members. Other preventative measures for the sick room could be made ahead of time to make the room ready before it is needed. Having all necessary items in the room will make for easy accessibility as well as containment of illness. Consider these 9 preventative measures:

1. All tissues, utensils, equipment, bedding, and clothing in contact with the sick person should be handled as if the germs of the illness were on them. Dishes and equipment should be washed in hot soapy water or wiped with 10% bleach or other disinfectant.
2. Use disposable dishes when possible so they can be discarded in plastic bags in the room.
3. Place all used tissues directly into a plastic bag that can be closed at the top before leaving the sick room. Have alcohol-based hand cleaning solution (Purell) at the bedside so the person can wash their hands after they cough or sneeze.
4. Gently fold or roll clothing and bedding into a plastic bag, being careful not to shake them, possibly releasing the germs into the air. Clothing and bedding should be washed in hot water.

5. Clean items in the room with a 10% bleach solution (made by combining 1 ounce of bleach with 9 ounces of water) or other disinfectant. Clean bathroom faucets and sink with 10% bleach or disinfectant wipes after the sick person has used them.
6. Wear a raincoat or other washable gown/coat over your clothes when in the room caring for the sick person. This gown will help to protect you from getting the germs on your clothes while caring for the person. This gown should stay in the room.
7. Wash your hands or use an alcohol-based cleaning solution (Purell) on your hands every time you leave the room. If disposable gloves are available, they can be worn while in the room but they should be removed in the room and discarded in the room, and then your hands must be washed.
8. Limit the people in close contact (within 6 feet) of the sick person. Keep the door to the sick room closed. Have a bell or cell phone by the bedside so the person can call for assistance when needed.
9. If respiratory masks (N95) are available, they should be worn by the sick person and the caretaker when they are in close contact.

Some items to consider when stocking a sick room are[41]:

- Bed with linens, pillow and blanket
- Small wastebasket or a bucket lined with a plastic garbage bag.
- Pitcher or large bottle for water
- Large plastic dishpan
- Clipboard with paper and a pen for writing in the daily log.
- Clock
- Hand crank or battery-powered radio
- Good source of light
- Flashlight with extra batteries
- A clothes hamper or a garbage can lined with a plastic garbage bag can be used to collect soiled clothing and bedding before they are washed.
- A bell or a noisemaker to call for assistance.
- Thermometer
- Tissues
- Hand wipes or a waterless hand sanitizer
- Cotton balls
- Rubbing alcohol, disinfectant or bleach
- Plastic garbage bags

41

https://www.storesonlinepro.com/files/2261183/uploaded/Checklist%20for%20Setting%20Up%20a%20Sick%20Room%20.pdf

- Measuring cup capable of holding 8 ounces or 250 ml
- Over-the-counter medications for use in the sick room
- Aprons or smocks (at least 2)
- Latex household cleaning gloves (2 pairs)
- Disposable vinyl gloves (2 boxes)
- Garbage bags
- N95 respirator masks (2 boxes) for use when the sick person is coughing or sneezing (can be purchased at hardware stores and some drugstores)

To prepare for longer-term scenarios, consider adding other medical supplies to the sick room. Further having some medical response packs pre-packaged cuts down on response time, and gives the caregiver more of an advantage in properly caring for the wounded. To prepare for a SHTF scenario, it would be beneficial to take into account the most likely medical situations you may come in contact with and plan accordingly. To conclude, preventing the transmission of an illness can be done with proper planning and preparation. A little forethought will help the caregiver be as efficient as possible in treating the ill patient, and in the process, keep the rest of household as healthy as possible.

25 Ways to Prevent Illness

By Daisy Luther

During any type of outbreak, you will hear you will hear in about 10,971 variations of the hit song "Big Pharma Will Save You." You'll be told that the "best way to prevent insert-disease-or-illness-of-the-month is to take your vaccine or prescription medication."

This is actually untrue.

The absolute, number one way to avoid contracting an illness is through social isolation. The second best way is through the exercise of good personal hygiene.

Follow these 25 tips to reduce the risk of contracting a communicable illness.

1. Wash your hands frequently when you are out.
2. Use a paper towel to open bathroom doors and turn on taps.
3. Although I'm normally not a big fan of hand sanitizer, use it during an outbreak if you have to touch things that everyone else has been touching, like the handle of the shopping cart, door knobs, and debit machines.

4. Use antibacterial wipes (or at least baby wipes) to wash your hands and wipe the steering wheel when you get back into your vehicle.
5. Avoid touching your face - this welcomes germs that are on your hands into your body.
6. Consider taking a quick shower and changing clothes when you return home, particularly if you have been in a germ-ridden place like a doctor's office or pharmacy.
7. Make sure the kids change clothes and thoroughly wash their hands when they return home from school.
8. I shouldn't really have to say this, but....wash your hands after using the bathroom and before preparing or eating food.

If your local area is being hit hard by an illness, practice avoidance to keep your family healthy.

9. Stay home as much as possible. (Obviously, if you have work and school outside the home, this become more difficult, but avoid malls, movie theaters, and sporting events for the duration of the epidemic.)
10. Stay away from sick people if you can.

11. Avoid eating at restaurants - you don't know the health or hygiene habits of the kitchen staff.

If someone in your family is sick, try to minimize the spread of the illness.

12. If you or a family member are sick, stay home from work or school to prevent passing it on to others.

13. If a family member is sick, keep them isolated away from the rest of the family.

14. Use antibacterial wipes to clean surfaces that the sick person touches - doorknobs, TV remotes, keyboards, toilet handles, and phones.

15. Immediate place dishes and flatware used by the sick person into hot, soapy dishwater with a drop of bleach in it.

16. Teach children to cough into the crook of their arm instead of covering their mouth with their hands.

17. Have the sick person wash their hands frequently with soap and water to help prevent spreading germs

through physical contact. If soap and water is unavailable, have them use hand sanitizer.

Some other ways to stay healthy are to use natural strategies to maximize your immune system. What's more, the healthier you are before a pandemic strikes, the more likely your own immune system will be to fight it off.

18. Drink lots of water to keep your system hydrated and efficient.

19. Take a high quality, organic multi-vitamin.

20. Take at least 3000 IUs of Vitamin D daily[42] - research has shown a link between a Vitamin D deficit and susceptibility[43] to the flu.

21. Eat lots of fruits and vegetables (preferably organic and pesticide free).

---

[42] http://articles.mercola.com/sites/articles/archive/2011/12/14/study-shows-vitamin-d-cuts-flu-by-nearly-50.aspx
[43] http://www.lewrockwell.com/2008/10/donald-w-miller-jr-md/dont-get-a-flu-shot-2/

22. Get 7-9 hours of sleep per day - a tired body has a weaker immunity against viruses.

23. Don't smoke - this weakens your resistance against respiratory illnesses and worsens the effect on your body if you do become ill.

24. Avoid or limit alcoholic beverages.

25. Avoid or limit processed foods.

Taking a Natural Approach to Pandemics

Excerpt from *The Prepper's Blueprint: The Step-by-Step Guide to Help You Prepare for Any Disaster*

By Tess Pennington

Herbal lore has it that, while the Plague was raging in France, a rash of burglaries of plague victims' homes was discovered. No effort was made, however, to apprehend the thieves, as it was assumed that they would soon succumb to the contagion in the homes they had robbed.

The thieves carried on their crime spree for some time, and people began to wonder why they had not become ill and die. It was then that the authorities began to pursue them... to discover the secret of their immunity to the Plague.

Once the burglars had been apprehended, they struck a bargain with the authorities that they should be set free in exchange for revealing the secret to their immunity to the Plague. It was then that the four thieves revealed the herbal disinfectant formula that rendered them immune to the Plague.

ALTERNATIVE FOUR THIEVES OIL
1 part eucalyptus
1 part rosemary
1 part cinnamon
1 part clove
1 part lemon
50 drops of a carrier oil (olive, jojoba, or your choice)

Put 50 drops of each oil in a 2 oz. bottle and then top it off with jojoba oil (I like jojoba oil because it seems to never go rancid).

APPLICATIONS:

- For personal protection, add a teaspoonful to bath water.
- Use as a topical spray for disinfecting surfaces and/or skin
- Apply 1-2 drops of Four Thieves on the bottoms of the feet and on the nape of the neck.
- Apply under the arms and on the chest.

FOUR THIEVES VINEGAR

Current theorists suggest that this formula, now called "Four Thieves Vinegar", may offer protection against fearsome possible threats, such as the flu, smallpox, and biological weapons, which concern us today, as all of its ingredients are either strong anti-bacterial agents, or have potent anti-viral properties.

This vinegar can be taken daily to ward off any potential pathogens, used in salads as a nutritious salad dressing or added to the bath water.

- 1 part lavender, dried
- 1 part sage, dried
- 1 part thyme, dried
- 1 part lemon balm (Melissa), dried
- 1 part hyssop, dried
- 1 part peppermint, dried
- 1 handful garlic cloves
- Raw (unpasteurized), organic apple cider vinegar

1. In a glass jar, place all dry ingredients.
2. Add raw (unpasteurized) organic apple cider vinegar and cover.
3. Set jar at room temperature for 6 weeks.

Homemade Electrolyte Replacement Powders

Sugar Option

2 quarts water
5-10 teaspoon of sugar
1 teaspoon of salt
1 teaspoon of baking soda
½ teaspoon of salt substitute (potassium salt)
1 pack of sugar-free drink flavoring

Sugar-Free Versions

Sugar free: Although adding sugar to your drink will help you keep your energy levels up, it's not a good option for everyone. People on a low-carb diet or people with diabetes, can choose a recipe that doesn't add sugar to the electrolyte drink:

Version 1

1 quart of water
2 tablespoons fresh lemon juice
3-4 tablespoons raw honey
¼ teaspoon of sea salt

Version 2

2 quarts of water
1 teaspoon of sea salt
1 teaspoon of baking soda
½ teaspoon of salt substitute (potassium salt)
1 pack of sugar free drink flavoring
Artificial sweetener to taste, optional

***

Part Three: Prepping for a Pandemic

Pandemic Preparedness

An excerpt from *The Prepper's Blueprint: The Step-by-Step Guide to Help You Prepare for Any Disaster*

By Tess Pennington

Tess Pennington has generously contributed the entire chapter on pandemic preparedness from her #1 best seller, *The Prepper's Blueprint: The Step-by-Step Guide to Help You Prepare for Any Disaster.* Tess's book is available exclusively on Amazon.

There are no exact death tolls for the 1918 Flu Pandemic (which actually came in 3 waves and lasted into well 1919). It was called the "greatest medical holocaust in history". Because of a rare shift of genetic material in the virus, no one had been able to build an immunity to the virus. The death toll was estimated at between 30 million and 50 million people worldwide. It moved so fast that within the first 6 months, 25 million people had caught the "Spanish Flu". More people died in one year of this flu than in the entire 4 years of the medieval "Black Plague." By turning into a vicious form of pneumonia, this strain of influenza killed people, often within hours of the first signs of illness.

The first confirmed outbreak in the United States occurred at an army base in Kansas. Within hours of the first reported illness, dozens of sick soldiers were in the infirmary. Within a week, more than 500 soldiers on that base had fallen ill. Meanwhile, 2 million troops were mobilized to Europe, where they introduced the deadly virus to France, England, Germany and Spain. One ship was not able to put out to sea because more than 10,000 soldiers on board were suffering from the virulent strain. More American soldiers died of the Spanish flu than deaths in combat in WWI, but what's more, they carried the flu with them as they shipped out all over the world.

So many people died at once that there was a shortage of morticians, coffins and gravediggers. Morgues were forced to stack bodies like "cordwood' in the hallways and mass graves were dug to try and deal with all of the corpses in an effort to prevent even more health risks. Public health ordinances were created to try to contain the pandemic, to little avail. Gauze masks were distributed, trains required a certificate of health before passengers were allowed to travel, and some towns required such certificates before a person could enter.

There are still no answers as to why this flu mutated and spread so quickly - as well, there are no answers on how to prevent such a thing from occurring again.

According to the Center for Disease Control[44] (CDC), serious, contagious disease outbreaks can and do happen. The CDC investigates new contagious diseases—averaging one new contagion per year. Given our vast array of transportation systems, modern society causes infectious disease to spread far more rapidly compared to any other time in recorded history; and because pandemics are fast moving, vaccines cannot be created fast enough to be of help.

Looking back at the Black Plague, those living in highly populated areas were hit hardest by this pandemic. The Black Death is estimated to have killed 30–60 percent of Europe's population.

When an outbreak occurs, those living in close proximity to others (especially in cities and high density population cities) will be more at risk. Pregnant women, infants, elderly people, or those with chronic medical conditions are at

---

44 http://www.pandemicflu.gov/news/contagion_outbreakcontrol.html

the highest risk and could be the first of the population to contract the contagious illness.

When the pandemic begins, many will remain in a state of denial about any approaching epidemic emergency and will not want to believe there will be long-lasting repercussions of such a disaster. When they begin to come out of their collective dazes, a widespread panic occurs, affecting everyone from citizens to city officials. Failure of adequate government response, population density, looters taking advantage of the high state of panic, and overwhelmed emergency medical response teams could all contribute to a societal breakdown[45].

Being prepared before the masses realize there is a problem will ensure that you can avoid the chaos as the hordes run to the store to stock up.

PREVENTION PLAYS A ROLE

Preventing the transmission of an illness rests in the hands of not only the individual, but the community as well. Prevention plays a very

---

[45] http://readynutrition.com/resources/the-anatomy-of-a-breakdown_12112012/

large role in preparing for a pandemic. There is a lot to be said for preventative measures.

As a whole, communities should take the necessary steps to be ready for potential challenges before a threat exists. Understand that areas where there are large numbers of people congregate (i.e., malls, schools, airports, grocery stores) pose the highest risk of spreading the epidemic more quickly. Breakdowns in communications, supply chains, payroll service issues, and healthcare staff shortages should be anticipated when preparing for a pandemic. To assist communities planning for a pandemic, the federal government has developed a Pandemic Severity Index. This index assists the government in gauging the severity of the epidemic based upon the amount of fatalities. Being familiar with the government's protocols before this type of emergency arises can help put you ahead of the game.

Some of the categories they use for determining their pandemic countermeasures are[46]:

- Covered Countermeasures
- Category of Disease
- Population

---

[46] http://www.flu.gov/

- Time period
- Geographic area
- Means of Distribution

If the government sees fit, they can activate pandemic mitigation measures. Some of these measures include the following:

1. Isolation and treatment (as appropriate) with influenza antiviral medications of all persons with confirmed or probable pandemic influenza. Isolation may occur in the home or healthcare setting, depending on the severity of the individual's illness and/or the current capacity of the healthcare infrastructure.
2. Voluntary home quarantine of members of households with confirmed or probable influenza case(s) and consideration of combining this intervention with the prophylactic use of antiviral medications, providing sufficient quantities of effective medications exist and that a feasible means of distributing them is in place.
3. Dismissal of students from schools (including public and private schools, as well as colleges and universities) and school-based activities and closure of childcare programs, coupled with protecting children and teenagers

through social distancing in the community to achieve reductions of out-of-school social contacts and community mixing.

4. Use of social distancing measures to reduce contact between adults in the community and workplace, including, for example, cancellation of large public gatherings and alteration of workplace environments and schedules to decrease social density and preserve a healthy workplace to the greatest extent possible without disrupting essential services. Enable institution of workplace leave policies that align incentives and facilitate adherence with the non-pharmaceutical interventions (NPIs) outlined above.

Source: www.flu.gov

My largest concern with pandemics is that supplies would be quickly exhausted, leaving many unprepared and ill-equipped to cope with the ordeal. This unpreparedness[47] will only fuel a more chaotic situation. These

---

[47] http://readynutrition.com/resources/the-unprepared-population-a-statistic-you-dont-want-to-be-a-part-of_11072013/

concerns are not new to most governments and steps have been taken to ensure communities are prepared and able to contain most epidemics.

The social distancing strategy mentioned above will occur through voluntary/involuntary home quarantine. If this occurs, the responsibility falls on our shoulders to ensure that we are able meet our needs. However, this is not anything new to a prepper.

INDIVIDUAL PREPARATION STARTS AT HOME

In the event of a pandemic, because of anticipated shortages of health care professionals and widespread implementation of social distancing techniques, it is expected that the large majority of individuals infected with the pandemic illness will be cared for in the home by family members, friends, and other members of the community who are not trained health care professionals. Persons who are more prone to contracting illnesses include those who are 65 years and older, children younger than five years old, pregnant women, and people of any age with certain chronic medical conditions or compromised immune systems.

HOW TO PREPARE FOR PANDEMICS

- Store a two week supply of water and food. During a pandemic, if you cannot get to a store, or if stores run out of inventory, it will be important for you to have extra supplies on hand.
- Have face masks to wear around those who may be ill or exposed to the illness.
- Periodically check your regular prescription drugs to ensure a continuous supply in your home.
- Have non-prescription drugs and other health supplies on hand, including pain relievers, stomach remedies, cough and cold medicines, fluids with electrolytes, and vitamins.
- Talk with family members and loved ones about how they would prefer to be cared for if they got sick
- Prepare a sick room for the home to limit family members' exposure to the virus. (See the supplemental section at the end of this chapter)
- Looters and crime waves can occur during this so ensure you have a means to protect yourself and your preps.

To decrease the chances of the virus spreading and infecting other household members as well as members of your community, it is important that every effort be made to limit exposure to the illness. Some considerations on how to prevent exposure to a pandemic outbreak are:

1. Avoid close contact with those who are ill.
2. Stay inside and avoid contact with others.
3. Avoid touching your mouth, nose and eyes during any pandemic.
4. Cover your mouth and nose with a tissue or your sleeve when coughing or sneezing. It may prevent those around you from getting sick.
5. Keep your hands clean. Washing your hands often will help protect you from germs. If soap and water are not available, use an alcohol-based hand rub or make your own natural hand sanitizer.
6. If you are ill, stay indoors or keep your distance from others.
7. Keep your immune system strong by getting lots of sleep, having a good diet and taking antioxidants and vitamins to protect your health.

ACTION ITEMS:

1.) Understand your community's role in pandemic preparedness. Find out ahead of time what your community's protocols are in the case of a sudden onset pandemic.

2.) For those with special needs, ensure that you have supplies ready for them (infants, elderly, handicapped, etc.).

3.) Plan accordingly for pets as well.

4.) Talk with family members and loved ones about how they would wish to be cared for if they became ill.

5.) Finding out your employer's plans and ask your child's school or day care what their protocol is during epidemic outbreaks.

6.) Have some supplies prepared in your workplace.

7.) Identify how you can get information, whether through local radio, TV, Internet or other sources.

Do you have the supplies you need to weather a pandemic?
By Daisy Luther

It's time to do a last minute check of your preps because by the time a general quarantine is announced in your area or you hear the mainstream suggesting that people should stay home, it will be too late to get the rest of your supplies. As well, at that point, the path of the pandemic will have progressed so much it will be unsafe to do so.

You need to be prepared to go into family lockdown mode for a minimum of 6 weeks should things get bad in your area, and preferably longer than that in the event that this takes a long time to contain. It's most likely that services such as public water and electricity will remain intact, but you should prepare as though they won't be[48], just in case.

Here's a quick checklist along with some links to resources. Base amounts on the number of family members you'll be sheltering.

---

[48] http://www.theorganicprepper.ca/the-big-blackout-why-im-going-low-tech-to-prep-for-an-emp-07302014

- Drinking water (1 gallon per person per day)
- Food (including items that don't require fuel for preparation)
- Heavy duty garbage bags
- Sanitation supplies such as toilet paper, paper towels, baby wipes, and feminine hygiene supplies)
- Entertainment - you'll want to be able to keep children and restless family members busy so get craft supplies, books, games, and puzzles
- Basic medical supplies
- Pandemic kits that contain protective clothing, including impermeable shoe covers, gowns, masks, and caps
- Extra N95 masks
- Nitrile gloves (high quality)
- Safety goggles with an elastic band to ensure a snug fit
- Antibacterial cleaners such as disposable wipes, bleach, and spray cleaners
- Antibacterial hand sanitizer

Note - we do not commonly use anti-bacterial products but in a situation like this, it's important to have this type of thing on hand in the event that there are issues with sanitation

If You're New to Prepping,

Start Here

By Daisy Luther

If you're new to preparedness, you may be reading some of the excellent and informative websites out there and feeling quite quite overwhelmed. While many sites recommend a one year supply of food, manual tools, and a bug out lodge in the forest, it's vital to realize that is a long-term goal, not a starting point.

A great starting point for someone who is just getting started on a preparedness journey is prepping specifically for a two-week power outage. If you can comfortably survive for two weeks without electricity, you will be in a far better position than most of the people in North America.

Even if you aren't convinced that hardcore preparedness is for you, it would still be difficult to argue against the possibility of a disaster lasting for a couple of weeks. Major natural disasters like Hurricane Sandy down to lesser storms like last year's Derecho in the Metro DC area are incontestable - storms happen and all you can do is be ready to weather them. As well, a large western US power company recently announced[49] that they did not foresee the ability to keep up with electrical demand this summer, and may institute rolling blackouts to cope with it. If you are prepared for two weeks without power, you are prepared for a wide range of short-term emergencies, including quarantines, interruptions of income, or civil unrest.

To prepare for a two week emergency, think about what you would need if the power went out and you couldn't leave your home for 14 days. Once you begin creating your plan, you may be surprised and discover that you already have most of what you need to batten down the hatches for a couple of weeks. It's just a matter of organizing it so you can see what you need.

Use the following information to create your personal 2 week preparedness plan. Modify the suggestions to adapt them to your particular home, family, and climate.

---

[49] http://www.thedailysheeple.com/north-american-electric-reliability-corporation-nerc-highlights-power-shortageses-for-several-states-this-summer_062013

Water

Everyone knows that clean drinking water is something you can't live without. In the event of a disaster, the water may not run from the taps, and if it does, it might not be safe to drink, depending on the situation. If there is a boil order in place, remember that if the power is out, boiling your water may not be as easy as turning on your stove.

Each family should store a two week supply of water. The rule of thumb for drinking water is 1 gallon per day, per person. Don't forget to stock water for your pets, also.

You can create your water supply very inexpensively. Many people use clean 2 liter soda pop bottles to store tap water. Others purchase the large 5 gallon jugs of filtered water from the grocery store. Consider a gravity fed water filtration device and water purification tablets as well.

Food and a way to prepare it

There are two schools of thought regarding food during a power outage. One: you need a cooking method that does not require the grid to be functioning. Two: you can store food that doesn't require cooking.

If you opt for a secondary cooking method, be sure that you have enough fuel for two weeks. Store foods that do not require long cooking times - for example, dried beans would use a great deal of fuel, but canned beans could be warmed up, or even eaten cold.

Heat (depending on your climate)

If your power outage takes place in the winter and you live in a colder climate, heat is another necessity. During the first 24 hours after a power outage, you can stay fairly warm if you block off one room of the house for everyone to group together in. Keep the door closed and keep a towel or blanket folded along the bottom of the door to conserve warmth. You can safely burn a couple of candles also, and in the enclosed space, your body heat will keep it relatively warm. As well, dress in layers and keep everything covered - wear a hat, gloves (fingerless ones allow you to still function), and a scarf.

However, after about 48 hours, that's not going to be enough in very cold weather. You will require back-up heat at this point in certain climates. If you are lucky enough to have a source of heat like a fireplace or woodstove, you'll be just fine as long as you have a supply of wood.

Consider a portable propane heater (and propane) or an oil heater. You have to be very careful what type of backup heat you plan on using, as many of them can cause carbon monoxide poisoning if used in a poorly ventilated area.

Sanitation needs

A common cause of illness, and even death, during a down-grid situation is lack of sanitation. We've discussed the importance of clean drinking water, but you won't want to use your drinking water to keep things clean or to flush the toilet.

For cleaning, reduce your need to wash things. Stock up on paper plates, paper towels, and disposable cups and flatware. Keep some disinfecting cleaning wipes and sprays (I don't recommend using antibacterial products on a regular basis, however in the event of an emergency they can help to keep you healthy.) Use hand sanitizer after using the bathroom and before handing food or beverages - there may be a lot more germs afoot in a disaster.

Look at your options for sanitation. Does your toilet still flush when the electricity is out? Many people discovered the hard way that the toilets didn't work when the sewage backed up in the high-rises in New York City in the aftermath of Hurricane Sandy. At our cabin, the toilet won't flush without power because the pump is electric.

If you are on a septic system, with no risk of the toilet backing up into the house, simply store some water for flushing in the bathroom. (At the first sign of a storm, we always fill the bathtub for this purpose.) Add the water to the tank so that you can flush.

If this is not an option, another solution is to stock up on extremely heavy duty garbage bags (like the kind that contractors use at construction sites) and kitty litter. Place a bag either in your drained toilet or in a bucket. Sprinkle some kitty litter in the bottom of the bag. Each time someone uses the bathroom, add another handful of litter. Be very careful that the bag doesn't get too heavy for you to handle it. Tie it up very securely and store it outside until services are restored.

Light

Lighting is absolutely vital, especially if there are children in the house. Nothing is more frightening than being completely in the dark during a stressful situation. Fortunately, it's one of the easiest things to plan for, as well as one of the least expensive.

Some lighting solutions are:

- Garden stake solar lights
- Candles
- Kerosene lamps

- Flashlights (don't forget batteries)
- Hand crank camping lantern
- Don't forget matches or lighters

Tools and supplies

Some basic items will make your life much easier during an emergency. Here are some things that are essential in the event of a power outage:

- Lighter/waterproof matches
- Batteries in various sizes
- Manual can opener
- Basic tools: Pliers, screwdriver, wrench, hammer
- Duct tape
- Crazy glue
- Sewing supplies
- Bungee cords

First Aid kit

It's important to have a basic first aid kit on hand at all times, but particularly in the event of an emergency. Your kit should include basic wound care items like bandages, antibiotic ointments, and sprays. As well, if you use them, keep on hand a supply of basic over-the-counter medications, like pain relief capsules, cold medicine, cough syrup, anti-nausea pills, and allergy medication. Particularly important if sanitation is a problem are anti-diarrheal medications.

Special needs

This is something that will be unique to every family. Consider the things that are needed on a daily basis in your household. It might be prescription medications, diapers, or special foods. If you have pets, you'll need supplies for them too. The best way to figure out what you need is to jot things down as you use them over the course of a week or so.

Part 4:
Supply Lists

Tess Pennington's 25 Must-Have Foods For Your Pantry

Stock up on the following items today to get your prepper pantry ready for the next extended emergency:

1. Canned fruits, vegetables, meats, and soups
2. Dried legumes (beans, lentils, peas)
3. Crackers
4. Nuts
5. Pasta sauce
6. Peanut butter
7. Pasta
8. Flour (white, whole wheat)
9. Seasonings (vanilla, salt, pepper, paprika, cinnamon, pepper, taco seasoning, etc.)
10. Sugar
11. Bouillon cubes or granules (chicken, vegetable, beef)
12. Kitchen staples (baking soda, baking powder, yeast, vinegar)
13. Honey
14. Unsweetened cocoa powder
15. Jell-O or pudding mixes
16. Whole grains (barley, bulgur, cornmeal, couscous, oats, quinoa, rice, wheat berries)
17. Nonfat dried milk
18. Plant-based oil (corn oil, vegetable oil, coconut oil, olive oil)

19. Cereals
20. Seeds for eating and sprouting
21. Popcorn (not the microwavable kind)
22. Instant potato flakes
23. Packaged meals (macaroni and cheese, hamburger helper, Ramen noodles, etc.)
24. Purified drinking water
25. Fruit juices, teas, coffee, drink mixes

Use the Food Storage Calculator at ReadyNutrition.com to help you determine how much food your family may need (http://readynutrition.com/resources/category /preparedness/calculators/)

Daisy Luther's No-Cook Food List

- Styrofoam plates
- Paper towels and napkins
- Plastic cutlery
- Baby wipes
- Disinfecting wipes
- Plastic cups
- Graham crackers with peanut butter
- Crackers with home canned cheese sauce
- Saltines with peanut butter
- Fresh fruit (apples, oranges, bananas)
- Canned juice
- Trail mix
- Dry cereal
- Cereal with milk
- Canned baked beans with ham
- Pretzels
- Nuts
- Pudding cups
- Canned fruit
- Jerky
- Pouches of pre-cooked and seasoned rice
- Cookies
- Granola bars
- Crackers

Dried Fruits: apricot, mango, banana, raisins, cranberries, pineapple
Sandwiches: Peanut butter and jelly, tuna, leftovers from the fridge, Nutella

Mac Slavo's Pandemic Supply List

- Drinking water (1 gallon per person per day)
- Food
- Sanitation supplies such as toilet paper, paper towels, baby wipes, and feminine hygiene supplies)
- Basic medical supplies and OTC medications
- Protective clothing
- Nitrile gloves
- Snug-fitting safety goggles
- Antibacterial cleaners such as disposable wipes, bleach, and spray cleaners

- Antibacterial hand sanitizer
- N-100 respirators (recommended by the World Health Organization)
- NATO SGE 400/3 Military Gas Mask (If going with such a mask, be sure to include some NBC filters.)
- Heavy Duty Plastic Sheeting to go over doors, windows or other potential airborne entry points (4 mm home coverall)
- Duct tape
- Portable toilet if one is not attached directly to the sick room.
- Disposable trash and toilet bags *Note: Waste must be disposed of properly because it may be contaminated*

Tess and Daisy's Home Medical Kit List

- Pain reliever (aspirin, acetaminophen, ibuprofen)
- Antacid
- Anti-diarrheal (Imodium)
- Anti-nausea (Dramamine)
- Cold medicine
- Allergy medication (Benadryl)
- Cough syrup
- Calamine lotion
- Hydrocortisone cream
- Antibacterial ointment
- Anbesol
- Clotrimazole (Monistat)
- Children's medications if applicable: stock children's versions of the above OTC medications
- First aid book
- Prescription medications (keep copies for records)
- Cold/flu medicines
- Vitamins
- Blood clotting
- Sterile gauze
- Dressing bandages
- Dressing rolls
- Medical tape
- Bandages of all sizes

- Alcohol wipes
- Hydrogen peroxide
- Witch hazel
- Cotton swabs
- Eye flushing solution (Saline solution for contact lens wearers works well)
- Anesthetic solution
- Hypodermic needles (for the antiseptic solution)
- Electrolyte tablets
- Scissors
- Tweezers
- Cold Packs
- Warm Blankets
- Antibiotic ointment
- Thermometers
- Skin irritation creams
- Gloves
- Mask
- Suture needles/string
- List of medical contact phone numbers
- Medical history file (if needed)

The Contributors

This collaboration would not be possible without the generosity of the following contributors:

Tess Pennington

Tess Pennington is the author of **The Prepper's Blueprint**, a comprehensive guide that uses real-life scenarios to help you prepare for any disaster. Because a crisis rarely stops with a triggering event the aftermath can spiral, having the capacity to cripple our normal ways of life. The well-rounded, multi-layered approach outlined in the **Blueprint** helps you make sense of a wide array of preparedness concepts through easily digestible action items and supply lists.

Tess is also the author of the highly rated **Prepper's Cookbook**, which helps you to create a plan for stocking, organizing and maintaining a proper emergency food supply and includes over 300 recipes for nutritious, delicious, life-saving meals.

Visit her web site, **ReadyNutrition.com,** for an extensive compilation of free information on preparedness, homesteading, and healthy living.

Mac Slavo

Mac Slavo is the founder of the popular **SHTFplan.com** community-based web site and is involved with various alternative media initiatives in an effort to promote awareness. His main areas of focus center around daily news, developing trends, preparedness information and community interaction.

Daisy Luther

Daisy Luther is a freelance writer and editor who lives in a small village in the Pacific Northwestern area of the United States. She is the author of **The Pantry Primer: How to Build a One Year Food Supply in Three Months**.

On her website, **TheOrganicPrepper.ca**, Daisy writes about healthy prepping, homesteading adventures, and the pursuit of liberty and food freedom. Daisy is a co-founder of the website **Nutritional Anarchy**, which focuses on resistance through food self-sufficiency.

Daisy's articles are widely republished throughout alternative media.

Lizzie Bennett

Lizzie Bennett retired from her job as a senior operating department practitioner in the UK earlier this year. Her field was trauma and accident and emergency and she has served on major catastrophe teams around the UK.

Lizzie publishes the website **UndergroundMedic.com** on the topic of preparedness.

Lisa Egan

Lisa Egan is a writer and editor who lives on the East Coast. She has a Bachelor of Science degree in Health Sciences with a minor in Nutrition and is a certified hypnotherapist.

Lisa has worked as a nutritionist and an American Council on Exercise personal trainer. She is a weight loss expert who takes a holistic approach to health and wellness. You can find Lisa's work on **NutritionalAnarchy.com, ReadyNutrition.com,** and **TheDailySheeple.com.**

Lily Dane

Lily Dane is a staff writer for The Daily Sheeple. Her goal is to help people to "Wake the Flock Up!"

Made in the USA
Charleston, SC
30 October 2014